Michelle Solórzano Ronquillo

Complications and Adverse Effects of Amphotericin B Use

Michelle Solórzano Ronquillo

Complications and Adverse Effects of Amphotericin B Use

In patients with HIV disease

ScienciaScripts

Imprint
Any brand names and product names mentioned in this book are subject to trademark, brand or patent protection and are trademarks or registered trademarks of their respective holders. The use of brand names, product names, common names, trade names, product descriptions etc. even without a particular marking in this work is in no way to be construed to mean that such names may be regarded as unrestricted in respect of trademark and brand protection legislation and could thus be used by anyone.

Cover image: www.ingimage.com

This book is a translation from the original published under ISBN 978-620-0-33148-9.

Publisher:
Sciencia Scripts
is a trademark of
Dodo Books Indian Ocean Ltd. and OmniScriptum S.R.L publishing group

120 High Road, East Finchley, London, N2 9ED, United Kingdom
Str. Armeneasca 28/1, office 1, Chisinau MD-2012, Republic of Moldova, Europe
Printed at: see last page
ISBN: 978-620-6-49506-2

DEDICATION

Dedicated to God above all for always giving me strength and encouragement to continue day by day.

To Reinaldo Solórzano Castaño and Carolina Ronquillo Vera for having been my faithful witnesses day and night of this long journey, for their unconditional support, for their infinite love and for their complete understanding in my days of family absence.

To my siblings, Reynaldo and Melissa, who are my greatest inspiration to keep going and to be the best example for them.

To Carmen Vera García, for all the times she gave me advice, for her care full of grandmotherly love, for always believing in me, Mamita Carmen.To Julia Castaño Rodríguez for her wise words "The best inheritance from a father is education". Always so right, this is for you too dear grandmother. To Ricardo Solórzano, this is also dedicated to you straight to heaven.

To the friends I met throughout my career, who today are like my brothers and sisters, for making this path the best of all, for the adventures, for the hours of study, for that and much more. Cinthia, Cristhian, Samantha, Andrés. And of course to my friends in life: Daniela, my comadre, and Macario, who have been part of this long journey.

Dedicated to all the people I love and who have an immense place in my life.

MICHELLE

THANK YOU

To my good teachers for having been a valuable pillar in my academic training.

To all the patients who, day after day, taught me more than just medicine; they were my best teachers of humanism and solidarity. Thank you for those pleasant talks full of personal experiences.

To our classmates who were undoubtedly a great support year after year.

MICHELLE

INDEX

COMPLICATIONS AND ADVERSE EFFECTS OF AMPHOTERICIN B USE IN PATIENTS WITH HIV DISEASE

SUMMARY

Introduction: Amphotericin B is a polyene antifungal agent with in vitro activity against a wide variety of fungal pathogens. The administration of amphotericin B can be associated with adverse effects after repeated administrations of the drug such as water and electrolyte disturbances, the most concerning toxicity and the one on which most studies have focused remains nephrotoxicity. This study aimed to determine adverse reactions to amphotericin B in patients with HIV/AIDS at the Hospital de Infectología de Guayaquil. Methodology: A descriptive, non-experimental study was carried out.

Results: Among HIV-positive patients, the most relevant fungal infection was cryptococcal meningoencephalitis (n=47;31.1%) and invasive aspergillosis (n=43;28.5%). In our study, the most frequently reported adverse reaction was nephrotoxicity (n=50;33.1%).

Keywords: Amphotericin B, HIV, Systemic Mycoses, Adverse Effects, Complications

INTRODUCTION

HIV/AIDS is a public health problem in the world, as well as in Ecuador, where there has been an increasing trend in the number of newly reported cases of HIV and AIDS, mainly in the last 10 years (1).

Since the original description in 1981 of an unusual cluster of cases of *Pneumocystis carinii pneumonia* and Kaposi's sarcoma in previously healthy men who have sex with men, substantial advances have been made in our understanding of acquired immunodeficiency syndrome (AIDS). The identification of a cytopathic retrovirus in 1983 and the development of a serological diagnostic test for human immunodeficiency virus (HIV) in 1985 have served as the basis for developing improvements in diagnosis. (2)

Amphotericin B is a polyene antifungal agent with in vitro activity against a wide variety of fungal pathogens. Despite the introduction of new antifungal agents for the treatment of systemic mycoses, amphotericin B remains the standard treatment for many severe invasive fungal infections. The administration of amphotericin B can be associated with immediate adverse effects, such as fever, chills, nausea, anaphylactic shock, arrhythmias, liver failure; adverse reactions occurring after repeated administrations of the drug such as water and electrolyte disturbances; the toxicity of most concern and on which most studies have focused remains nephrotoxicity. (3)

In our country there has not been a study in which adverse drug reactions to amphotericin B have been determined; The drug is available in several of its presentations, no reviews on efficacy or adverse reactions have been observed, on this basis it was proposed to find out why this compound is indicated, how it is used, what adverse reactions are observed, the outcome in a group of patients with HIV/AIDS, it is proposed to conduct a retrospective, descriptive study with the universe of APPS patients treated with amphotericin B for systemic fungal disease, especially meningeal cryptococcosis. The respective research variables were carried out with the aim of interpreting and determining the adverse reactions of this type of patient, regardless of the outcome of the treatment that each individual received.

CHAPTER I

- THE PROBLEM

.1 PROBLEM STATEMENT

Amphotericin B is considered the treatment of choice for severe fungal infections. However, its administration is associated with adverse reactions, mainly nephrotoxicity, which sometimes hinder its use. Incorporation of amphotericin B into lipid infusions has been reported to decrease its toxicity, but the reason for this phenomenon has not been fully elucidated. It has been suggested that this effect may be due to the slowing of the passage of amphotericin B into tissues (4).

The increase in recent years of immunosuppressed patients and diseases requiring the use of cytotoxic or immunosuppressive drugs has increased the incidence of serious fungal infections, leading to the need to test the effectiveness and toxicity of treatment. Amphotericin B is the broadest spectrum antifungal available to date and can be used for most fungal infections (5).

Adverse drug reactions (ADRs) are among the top ten causes of morbidity and mortality worldwide. Meta-analyses show 9.5% of ADRs for hospitalised children and 2.4% as a reason for admission. Children are a particularly susceptible population for ADRs; factors include the pharmacokinetic differences that occur in children and the fact that they are more susceptible to ADRs.

observed at different stages of growth and development, plasma levels of the drug achieved in different pathologies and physiological immaturity (5).

Amphotericin B (AnB) is the most commonly used antifungal for the treatment of opportunistic mycoses, especially in severe patients. Many of the ADRs observed with the use of this antifungal are due to misuse of the drug. Among the best known ADRs are fever, nausea, vomiting, thrombophlebitis, myalgia, nephrotoxicity with proteinuria, cylindruria, renal tubular acidosis and hypokalaemia. In addition, anaemia, white blood cell and megakaryocyte depression may occur after prolonged periods of administration (6).

.2 PROBLEM FORMULATION

What are the adverse reactions that have occurred in patients with HIV/AIDS treated with amphotericin B during the period 2015 - 2017 in patients of the Hospital de Infecto logia de Guayaquil?

What is the incidence of adverse events due to the use of amphotericin B in HIV/AIDS patients at the Infectious Diseases Hospital in the city of Guayaquil?

What is the prevalence of amphotericin B use in hospitalised patients at the Infectious Diseases hospital in Guayaquil?

.3 GENERAL AND SPECIFIC OBJECTIVES

General Objective

To determine the incidence of complications and adverse reactions due to the use of amphotericin B in patients with HIV/AIDS in the Hospital de Infectología de Guayaquil from 2015 to 2017.

Specific Objectives

To establish the staging of HIV/AIDS patients who experienced adverse reactions during treatment with amphotericin B.

To analyse the incidence of amphotericin B use in HIV/AIDS patients at the Infectious Diseases Hospital in Guayaquil.

.4 JUSTIFICATION OF THE PROBLEM

The purpose and importance of this study is to assess the frequency, incidence, clinical and epidemiological characteristics of patients with HIV/AIDS who were treated with amphotericin B and developed complications during the period 2016 - 2018 in the Daniel Rodríguez Maridueña Hospital, since local information on this type of adverse events is relatively scarce, this study is conducted to correlate the figures of new cases with previous studies and statistical data from this institution, to focus on the prevention and reduction of their frequency. Data will be taken as research variables based on clinical manifestations, general condition of patients, viral load, CD4 lymphocyte count, type of mycosis, days of antibiotic therapy and recording of adverse reactions.

.5 DELIMITATION

The research work was carried out at the Daniel Rodríguez Maridueña Hospital, "Infectious Diseases" in the city of Guayaquil, from 2015 to 2017.

.6 VARIABLES

VARIABLES	CONCEPT	DIMENSION	INDICATOR	SCALE VALUATION	SOURCE
Age	Time elapsed from birth to the date of implementation of the study.	Chronological age	Years Compliments	Quantitative a Discreet	History Clinic
Sex	Category to classify people according to their sexual characteristics.	Phenotypic, if the person recording the information is the one who assigns the sex to the person under investigation on the basis of secondary sexual characteristics.	Phenotype	Qualitative Dichotomous	History Clinic

Adverse drug reactions as	Any response to a medicinal product that is noxious and unintended, and that occurs at doses normally used in humans for prophylaxis, diagnosis or treatment of disease.	Nephro-toxicity Hepato-toxicity Water and electrolyte disorders Spinal/hematopoietic disorders	Type of Adverse drug reaction to	Qualitative Nominal	History Clinic
Stay Hospital	Period during which the patient remains in hospital.	In this case, length of stay is treated as a simple variable and does not need to be disaggregated into dimensions such as pre-surgical, post-surgical, scheduled or unscheduled stay.	Days of hospitalisation	Quantitative Discreet	History Clinic

.7 HYPOTHESIS

Adverse events and complications secondary to amphotericin B administration in HIV-infected patients are correlated to the form of administration and days of administration, and may also be related to age, associated fungal infection and sex of the patient.

CHAPTER II

- THEORETICAL FRAMEWORK

.1 HISTORY

During the second half of the 20th century, the incidence of complicated and invasive fungal infections increased in certain types of immunocompromised patients. As for example in critically ill neutropenic patients, increasing morbidity and mortality, the use of amphotericin B has been a mainstay in the treatment of this type of infection, despite its long history and potentially life-saving therapy, there is reluctance to its indication mainly due to the frequent occurrence of adverse reactions. (6)

Amphotericin B was marketed during the 1950s and its use is not without toxicity. Despite years of clinical experience in the management of this drug, until the mid-1990s there was still controversy about the available forms of administration, dosage regimen and duration of therapy that would allow for greater efficacy in clinical therapy with a lower risk of adverse effects and toxicity (6).

The various forms of administration of AnB in lipid formulations, marketed since the second half of the 1990s, have improved the optimisation of therapy in clinical practice.

as their administration has been shown to be associated with a lower incidence of adverse reactions (7).

Amphotericin B during the 1950s; due to the lack of availability of forms of administration in lipid emulsions and liposomes, the use of AnB in an excipient with lipophilic characteristics such as Intralipid 20 was frequent, as stability studies were not available to show how long it could be preserved before use (7).

.2 ORIGIN AND CHEMICAL STRUCTURE

Amphotericin B is produced by the actinomycete Streptomyces nodosus. It is a heptaene macrolide. The molecule consists of a hydrophilic portion of several hydroxylated carbons, a hydrophobic portion consisting of seven carbon atoms linked by double bonds (polyene) and a mycosamine side chain which is an aminodeoxyhexose. (6)

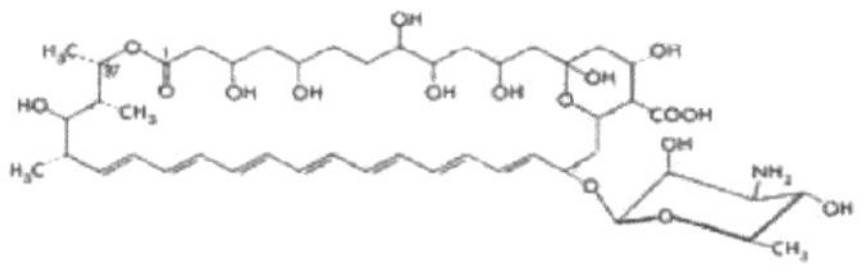

Anfotericina B

According to Catalán in 2015, amphotericin B can behave as a fungistatic or fungicide depending on the sensitivity of the fungus and the concentration reached at the site of infection. In the conventional formulation (amphotericin B deoxycholate) [ABD], sodium deoxycholate and sodium phosphate are used as excipient. Amphotericin B lipid complex [ABCL] is a lipid-associated formulation of amphotericin B (L-a-dimyristophosphatidylcholine; L-a-dimyristophosphatidylglycerol; L-a-dimyristophosphatidylglyceroly amphotericin B) and liposomal amphotericin B [ABL] is a compound of hydrogenated soy phosphatidylcholine, cholesterol, di-tearoylphosphatidylglycerol and amphotericin B. (4)

.3 MECHANISM OF ACTION

Gonzalez et al. indicated that Anf-B binds avidly to membrane sterols of eukaryotic cells, but not of prokaryotes. It has a higher affinity for ergosterol in fungi than for cholesterol in mammalian cells. As a consequence of this binding, alterations in membrane structure occur, probably due to the formation of pores composed of small aggregates of amphotericin B and sterols. These defects result in membrane depolarisation and increased permeability for protons and monovalent cations. The cellular effects of amphotericin depend on a number of factors such as the growth phase of the cells; dosage and the way the drug is administered. The main mechanism of action is through binding to the ergosterol of the fungal cell membrane. This binding allows the formation of pores and the release of electrolytes, resulting in the formation of pores and the release of electrolytes.

cell lysis. The drug also binds to cholesterol in mammalian cells, which may account for some of its toxicity. AnB also causes oxidative damage and inhibition of fungal cell metabolic activity (3).

.4 ANTIFUNGAL SPECTRUM

It has a broad spectrum. It is active against Aspergillus s p p p., Blastomyces dermatiti dis, Candida s p p p., Coccidioides immitis, Cryptococcus neoformans, Histoplasma capsulatum and Paracoccidioides brasiliensis. It is also effective against Absidia s p p p., Mucor spp. and Rhizopus spp. and those susceptible species of the genera Conidiobolus, Basiodiobolus and Sporothrix. Exceptions are some C a n d i d a species such as Candida lusitaniae, Candida guilliermondii, Candida lipolytica or Candida tropicalis; Pseudalescheria boydii and some strains of Fusarium and Trichosporon show clinical resistance and/or high minimum inhibitory concentrations (MIC) to this drug (3).

.5 PHARMACOKINETIC AND PHARMACODYNAMIC CHARACTERISTICS

Oral absorption is minimal (5%), so the route of administration of choice for IFI treatment is intravenous (iv). They are extensively bound to plasma lipoproteins (90-95%). The volume of distribution (Vd) is high at 4l/kg.

It reaches high concentrations in liver, spleen, lung and kidneys. In pleural fluid, peritoneal fluid, synovial fluid and aqueous humour, concentrations of the drug are 50-

60% of the minimum plasma concentration. It penetrates poorly into cerebrospinal fluid (CSF) (24%), increasing in cases of meningeal inflammation. It crosses the placenta well. There are no clinical trials available to determine elimination in human milk or safety in pregnant women (8).

It is partially metabolised in the liver and eliminated in bile (<15%) and 45% in urine. The initial elimination half-life is 24 h followed by a slower terminal elimination of about 15 days. Due to low renal elimination, no dosage adjustment is necessary in renal failure (RF), haemodialysis (HD) or peritoneal dialysis (PD). No dosage adjustment is necessary in hepatic insufficiency (LH). (8)

Torrado et al. in a 2015 study suggest that, in terms of absorption, AnB is a drug that is practically not absorbed orally (only 5% of the administered dose is detected) and is normally used by this route for topical and localised use in the infection.

Regarding the other routes of administration, intramuscular administration is very irritating and is not administered in this way. For the treatment of systemic infections, it should be administered intravenously in the different formulations: conventional (AnB-C) and lipid (ABCL, AnB-L) diluted in 5% glucose serum, so that the bioavailability of AnB is 100% (5).

In its distribution, conventional AnB is widely distributed in different tissues; only 10% of the dose remains in plasma. Its volume of distribution is approximately 4L/kg, reflecting the wide tissue distribution of the drug. It accumulates primarily in the liver, kidney, lung, heart, muscle and adrenal glands. It binds strongly to proteins (90-95%), mainly beta-lipoproteins, erythrocytes and plasma cholesterol. AnB hardly crosses the blood-brain barrier, with very low concentrations found in cerebrospinal fluid (2-4% of serum concentrations); it also penetrates little into other biological fluids. (5)

Renal excretion of unmetabolised AnB varies from 3% to 5% (detectable 24 hours after administration and in bile from 0.8% to 14% of the daily dose administered, so there is no need to modify the dose in patients with renal or hepatic failure. About 60% of the elimination metabolism of AnB is not established, although studies have been carried out to better understand this metabolism, and a number of unidentified metabolisation products have been found, which may be the result of probable hepatic metabolism.

.6 ADVERSE REACTIONS AND TOXICITY

Hepatotoxicity: Hepatotoxicity is defined as liver injury or damage caused by exposure to a drug or other non-pharmacological agents. The term adverse drug reaction refers to the occurrence of unintended deleterious effects that occur with drug doses used for prophylactic and therapeutic purposes. These adverse reactions affecting the liver are more difficult to define, so the concept has been established by consensus meetings and includes increased alanine aminotransferase greater than twice the upper limit of normal; increased serum direct bilirubin concentration greater than twice the upper limit of normal; or increased aspartate aminotransferase, alkaline phosphatase and total bilirubin concentration, provided that one of them exceeds more than twice the upper limit of normal. (9)

Nephrotoxicity: This is defined as injury to the kidneys, which can be caused by drugs or substances that are harmful to the organism; the main alterations that occur in the kidney can be classified according to their histopathology, into interstitial tubular injury, glomerular injury and vascular injury, which will have different clinical manifestations according to the region of the kidney that is altered (10).

Medullary Toxicity: Drug-induced agranulocytosis is a rare and serious adverse reaction, which can be caused by a variety of drugs. The diagnosis of this reaction requires a high degree of suspicion and the fulfilment of well-established diagnostic criteria. It is considered a serious, life-threatening haematological disorder with a mortality of 3-8%. It is characterised by a severe and selective reduction of circulating neutrophils, the red and megakaryocytic series may also be affected (11).

Schaffner et al. in 2015 in their study on the administration of ampho-B found that the incidence of adverse reactions to ABD treatment is high. Two types of adverse reactions can be considered: a. Immediate: in most patients, fever, chills and tremors are very common during the infusion of the drug in the first week. Sometimes accompanied by headache, vomiting and hypotension. These effects can be reduced by prior administration of antipyretics, antihistamines and/or antiemetics (12).

In relation to dose and/or duration of treatment: the most relevant adverse effect and the main limiting factor for its use is nephrotoxicity. Renal damage is usually reversible upon discontinuation of the drug, although it may take several weeks to normalise. Nephrotoxicity can be reduced by ensuring adequate hydration of the patient. More than 25% of patients develop hypokalaemia and hypomagnesaemia.

More than 25% of patients develop hypokalaemia and hypomagnesaemia. Normocytic normochromic anaemia frequently develops as a consequence of inhibition of erythropoietin synthesis and also by direct action on the bone marrow. Association with leukopenia and thrombopenia is rare. Thrombophlebitis associated with peripheral administration of ABD is frequent. Extravasation of the drug can lead to tissue necrosis. Anaphylactic reactions are very rare (12).

According to Torrado et al. the rapid administration of the drug (in less than 60 min) intravenously can trigger cardiac arrhythmias and cardiac arrest. Intrathecally it can cause nausea, vomiting, headache, urinary retention, headache, radiculitis, paresis, paraesthesia, visual disturbances and chemical meningitis. Monitoring of serum potassium and magnesium levels is always advisable due to the tendency to hypokalaemia and hypomagnesaemia with this type of drug (5).

The frequency of significant renal damage defined as a 50% decrease in glomerular filtration rate and a creatinine equal to or greater than 2mg/dl is approximately 30%, but the reported incidence is variable as various definitions are used. Renal toxicity occurs more frequently in men, in those over 65 years of age, depending on the underlying disease, particularly if haematopoietic cell transplantation has been performed, if other nephrotoxic drugs are used concomitantly and with cumulative dosing.

.7 INFECTION BY CRYPTOCOCCUS NEOFORMANS IN HIV/AIDS PATIENTS

Although cryptococcal infection begins in the lungs, meningitis is the most frequent manifestation of cryptococcosis among people with advanced immunosuppression. However, the infection is more properly characterised as "meningoencephalitis" rather than meningitis, as the brain parenchyma is almost always involved on histological examination. (13)

.8 EPIDEMIOLOGY

The vast majority of cases of cryptococcal meningoencephalitis are seen in patients with AIDS and a CD4 count <100 cells/microL. Patients with cryptococcosis may not receive antiretroviral therapy (ART) or may receive ART but have drug resistance or poor adherence to their prescribed regimen (14).

In 2008, it was estimated that approximately 957,900 cases of cryptococcal meningoencephalitis occurred worldwide each year, resulting in more than 600,000 deaths. The regions with the highest number of estimated cases in 2006 were sub-Saharan Africa (720,000 cases; range, 144,000 to 1.3 million), followed by South and Southeast Asia (120,000 cases; range, 24,000 to 216,000) (1).

The incidence of cryptococcal meningoencephalitis has declined with the widespread availability of antiretroviral drugs, with an estimated 223,100 cases per year worldwide, resulting in 181,100 deaths per year in 2014. However, cryptococcal disease remains a leading cause of mortality in developing countries, where access to ART is limited and HIV prevalence remains high. (15)

Early diagnosis and treatment can help reduce mortality related to cryptococcal meningitis. One way to diagnose cryptococcal infection early in the course of the disease is through detection of serum cryptococcal antigen (CrAg), which can be detected at least three weeks before the onset of neurological symptoms.

.9 CLINICAL MANIFESTATIONS

Symptoms of cryptococcal meningoencephalitis usually begin indolently over a period of one to two weeks. The most common symptoms are fever, malaise and headache. Stiff neck, photophobia and vomiting are seen in a quarter to a third of patients. Occasionally, patients may present with coma and fulminant death within days. Other symptoms suggestive of disseminated disease include cough, dyspnoea and rash (16).

Initial physical examination may be notable for lethargy or confusion in association with fever. In one report, 24 percent of patients had alterations in presentation and 6 percent had focal neurological deficits, such as cranial neuropathies. Other manifestations of disseminated disease may be evident, including tachypnoea and skin lesions resembling molluscum contagiosum. Increased diastolic hypertension may reflect increased intracranial pressure (17).

General laboratory studies are non-specific. Patients with advanced immunosuppression may have leukopenia, anaemia, hypoalbuminaemia and an increased fraction of gamma globulin antibodies. (17)

.10 DIAGNOSTICS

We have a high index of suspicion for cryptococcal meningoencephalitis in patients with advanced HIV infection (CD4 cell count <100 cells/microL) who have isolated fever and headache. Initial evaluation includes a careful history, neurological examination and serum cryptococcal antigen (CrAg). Evaluation should also include a lumbar puncture (LP) to assess for increased intracranial pressure and cerebrospinal fluid (CSF) culture to confirm the diagnosis in those with symptoms and/or a positive serum CrAg. (18)

.11 IMAGING AND RADIOLOGY

Prior to LP, patients suspected of having massive intracranial pressure and/or central nervous system (CNS) mass lesions should have neuroimaging (e.g., computed tomography [CT] or magnetic resonance imaging [MRI]). A detailed discussion on when to perform neuroimaging prior to LP is found elsewhere.

Imaging can detect the presence of mass lesions, increased intracranial pressure and/or hydrocephalus, all of which affect treatment decisions.

Imaging may suggest a possible increase in ICP with or without space-occupying lesions/mass in patients with cryptococcal meningoencephalitis. While LP and CSF removal may be beneficial for both diagnostic and therapeutic purposes, the risks and benefits of the procedure should be discussed with the patient and/or health care proxy, given the very small but possible possibility of brain herniation in the setting of elevated intracranial pressure. Mass lesions due to *C. neoformans* are rarely seen in patients with HIV infection; they are more common with *C. gattii* infections (18).

.12 CULTIVATION AND MICROBIOLOGY

A lumbar puncture (LP) is necessary to obtain CSF for confirmatory testing to make the diagnosis of cryptococcal meningoencephalitis. The CSF profile classically shows a low CSF white blood cell count (e.g. <50 cells/microL) with a mononuclear predominance.

CSF should be sent for cryptococcal culture; cream-coloured mucoid colonies are usually seen on agar plates within three to seven days. Since the burden of organisms is usually high in AIDS patients, an India ink preparation of CSF generally shows typical round encapsulated yeast organisms compatible with cryptococcus in 60 to 80 percent of patients.

Cryptococcal antigen (CrAg) can be detected in serum and CSF by immunodiagnostic techniques such as latex agglutination or enzyme-linked immunosorbent sandwich assay (ELISA). The lateral flow assay (LFA) is an alternative approach to detect cryptococcal antigen. It is a simple dipstick test that is inexpensive to perform and can be used on urine, blood, serum, CSF or plasma samples.

In AIDS patients with suspected cryptococcal meningoencephalitis, the sensitivity of serum CrAg testing is comparable to CSF testing and is a useful diagnostic modality in patients who cannot undergo lumbar puncture. CrAg titres generally correlate with body burden and prognosis. As an example, with the use of pre-emptive serum CrAg screening in asymptomatic AIDS patients, a titre of >1: 160 predicted the presence of CNS involvement.

Cryptococcal PCR for CNS infections (e.g. BioFire FilmArray), which screens for the presence of *C. neoformans* and *C. gattii,* is increasingly being used in clinical practice. In a study from Africa, this test detected cryptococcus in the CSF of patients diagnosed with a first episode of cryptococcal infection with a sensitivity and specificity >90 per cent, and was used to help distinguish a persistent infection from an immune reconstitution inflammatory syndrome (IRIS). (1)

.13 ANTIFUNGAL THERAPY

The main antifungal agents used for the treatment of cryptococcal meningoencephalitis include intravenous amphotericin B, oral flucytosine and oral fluconazole. Intrathecal or intraventricular amphotericin B is not recommended as systemic administration demonstrates good efficacy and these other direct routes may be associated with arachnoiditis.

For induction therapy we recommend liposomal amphotericin B (3 to 4 mg/kg intravenously [IV] per day) plus flucytosine (100 mg/kg per day orally in four divided doses). Induction therapy should be administered for at least two weeks. The duration should be extended if clinical improvement is not observed and/or if CSF sterilisation has not yet been achieved (19).

Amphotericin B deoxycholate is frequently associated with electrolyte disturbances, anaemia, renal failure and infusion site reactions such as drug fever and rigors. These adverse events are reduced when liposomal preparations are used. The risk of renal dysfunction associated with amphotericin B may be reduced by infusion of normal saline before and during therapy. (19)

CHAPTER III

- METHODOLOGICAL FRAMEWORK

.1 METHODOLOGY

This is a non-experimental research, with observational and descriptive analysis, for which we used as a source of information a database of patients under the ICD-10 codes B-24, B451, B-450, B457, corresponding to Human Immunodeficiency Virus Infection, cerebral, pulmonary and disseminated cryptococcosis, provided by the Department of Statistics of the Infectious Diseases Hospital of the City of Guayaquil "José Daniel Rodríguez Maridueña", which contained the medical record numbers of all patients who were evolved under this code in the TICS System, a system used by the health entities that form part of the care network of the Ministry of Public Health of Ecuador, which contained the laboratory reports and echocardiographies of the patients attended during the study period.

.2 CHARACTERISATION OF THE WORKING AREA

The research is carried out at the Hospital de Infectología de Guayaquil "José Rodríguez Maridueña", Guayaquil Province, Ecuador.

.3 UNIVERSE AND SAMPLE

The universe consists of all patients admitted to the Daniel Rodríguez Maridueña

HIV/AIDS Hospital with systemic and severe mycosis treated with amphotericin B who developed complications and adverse reactions during the study period, which runs from January 2016 to December 2018. The sample will consist of patients who meet the inclusion criteria.

.4 INCLUSION CRITERIA

- Patients with HIV/AIDS who presented with severe or systemic mycosis and whose treatment included the use of AnB with the development of adverse events.
- Patients over 18 years of age

.5 EXCLUSION CRITERIA

- Patients with HIV/AIDS who developed systemic mycoses and were treated with other antifungals except AnB.
- Causes of other diseases or pathologies that have produced disturbances and adverse reactions

.6 FEASIBILITY

The present study is feasible, as it represents an interest in the public health area of the country, as PLWHA patients have disseminated fungal infections that are difficult to treat with antimicrobials that can produce adverse reactions and complicate the patient's condition.

This research work has all the necessary permissions for data collection, provided by the Infectious Diseases Hospital, and subsequent statistical analysis and reporting of results.

.7 TYPE OF RESEARCH

Descriptive research

.8 HUMAN AND PHYSICAL RESOURCES

Human resources

- Researcher
- Tutor

Material Resources.

- HP Computer
- EPSON 320 Printer
- Bonds paper sheets
- Printer cartridge
- Biros
- Notebook

- Capetas Manila with headband
- Charcoal pencil 26
- Draft.
- Medical records
- Complications and Epicrisis Report

.9 VARIABLES

VARIABLES	CONCEPT	DIMENSION	INDICATOR	SCALE VALUATION	SOURCE
Age	Time elapsed from birth to the date of implementation of the study.	Chronological age	Years Compliments	Quantitative a Discreet	History Clinic
Sex	Category to classify people according to their sexual characteristics.	Phenotypic, if the person recording the information is the one who assigns the sex to the person under investigation on the basis of secondary sexual characteristics.	Phenotype	Qualitative Dichotomous	History Clinic

Adverse drug reactions	Any response to a medicinal product that is noxious and unintended, occurring at doses normally used in humans for prophylaxis, diagnosis or treatment of disease.	Nephro-toxicity Hepato-toxicity Water and electrolyte disorders Spinal/haemato-poietic disorder	Type of Adverse drug reaction to	Qualitative Nominal	History Clinic
Stay Hospital	Period during which the patient remains in hospital.	In these cases the length of stay is treated as a simple variable and does not need to be disaggregated into dimensions such as pre-surgical, post-surgical, scheduled or unscheduled stay.	Days of hospitalisation	Quantitative Discreet	History Clinic

.10 EVALUATION OR DATA COLLECTION INSTRUMENTS

The identification of HIV/AIDS patients with systemic and severe mycosis treated with amphotericin B who developed complications and adverse reactions in Guayaquil in the study period, during the period 2015 - 2017; The required information was obtained from the review of the medical records of patients who met the inclusion criteria, the data were collected on a data collection sheet prepared by the researcher and the information collected was used to create a database in Microsoft Excel and the IBM - SPSS programme for the preparation of tables and bar graphs representing the variables of the study.

.11 METHODOLOGY FOR THE ANALYSIS OF RESULTS

Frequency tables and bar charts were used to show the incidence of adverse reactions in the study group. Contingency tables or cross-tabulations were used to show the correlation between 2 variables. Measures and characteristics of the study population were used, qualitative variables such as gender, type of mycosis, complications, and numerical measures for quantitative variables.

.12 BIOETHICAL CONSIDERATIONS

Since this was a descriptive study and in compliance with the Bioethics standards related to the principles of: autonomy, beneficence, confidentiality and justice, the Teaching and Research Department of the Daniel Rodríguez

Maridueña Hospital was consulted for the respective approval of the study. In addition, the integrity of the patients was respected, ensuring the confidentiality of all personal information collected from the medical records.

CHAPTER IV

- RESULTS

.1 ADVERSE REACTIONS IN SYSTEMIC MYCOSIS/VIH PATIENTS TREATED WITH ANF-B HOSPITAL OF INFECTIOUS DISEASES PERIOD 2015 - 2017

		Frequency	Percentage	Percentage valid	Cumulative percentage
Valid	HYPERKALIEMIA	18	11,9	11,9	11,9
	HYPONATHROMIA	16	10,6	10,6	22,5
	ACUTE LIVER FAILURE	45	29,8	29,8	52,3
	NEPHROTOXICITY	50	33,1	33,1	85,4
	NOT REGISTERED	22	14,6	14,6	100,0
	Total	151	100,0	100,0	

Table 1 ADVERSE REACTIONS IN SYSTEMIC MYCOSIS/HIV PATIENTS TREATED WITH ANF-B HOSPITAL OF INFECTOLOGY PERIOD 2015 - 2017 SOURCE: DEPARTMENT OF STATISTICS OF THE HOSPITAL OF INFECTOLOGY AUTHOR: MICHELLE SOLÓRZANO RONQUILLO

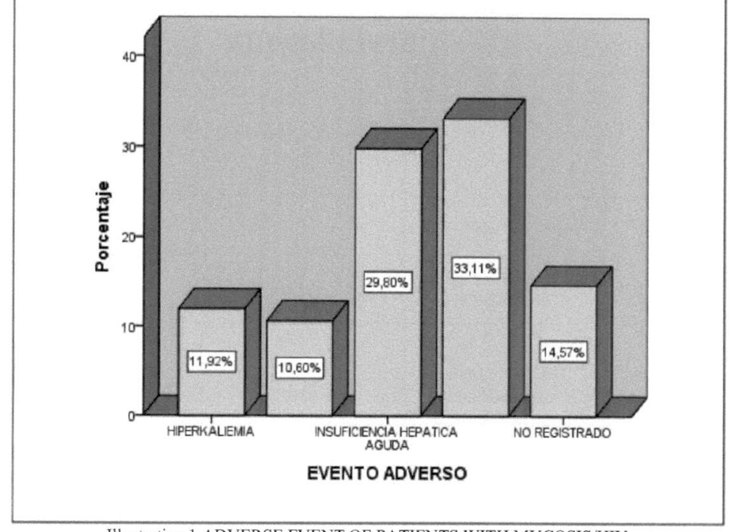

Illustration 1 ADVERSE EVENT OF PATIENTS WITH MYCOSIS/HIV
INFECTOLOGY HOSPITAL
PERIOD 2015 - 2017

Analysis: Administration of amphotericin B can be associated with adverse effects that occur after repeated administrations of the drug, including hypohyperkalemia, bone marrow toxicity, nephrotoxicity, in our patient group we can identify that there is a high incidence of nephrotoxicity (33,1%) in patients receiving amphotericin B in the treatment of systemic mycosis in HIV patients, acute liver failure data recorded with increased prothrombin time in 29.8% of patients, electrolyte disturbances of potassium (11.9%) and sodium (10.6%) of all patients.

.2 SYSTEMIC MYCOSIS REGISTRY/VIH HOSPITAL OF INFECTIOUS DISEASES PERIOD 2015 - 2017

MYCOSIS/HIV

		Frequency	Percentage	Percentage valid	Cumulative percentage
Valid	INVASIVE ASPERGILLOSIS	43	28,5	28,5	28,5
	DISSEMINATED CANDIDIASIS	5	3,3	3,3	31,8
	CRYPTOCOCOSIS DISEMINATED	47	31,1	31,1	62,9
	HISTOPLASMOSIS	9	6,0	6,0	68,9
	MENINGOENCEPHALITIS CRIPTOCOCICA	47	31,1	31,1	100,0
	Total	151	100,0	100,0	

Table 2 MYCOSIS/HIV INFECTOLOGY HOSPITAL YEAR 2015 - 2017
SOURCE: STATISTICS DEPARTMENT OF THE INFECTIOUS DISEASES HOSPITAL
AUTHOR. IRM. MICHELLE SOLÓRZANO RONQUILLO

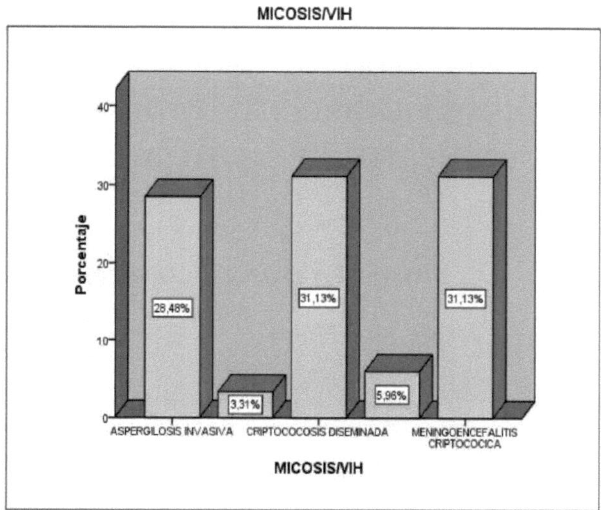

Illustration 2 MYCOSIS/HIV INFECTOLOGY HOSPITAL YEAR 2015 - 2017

Analysis: Most acute infections are asymptomatic or mild and remain undiagnosed. Typical manifestations are fever, headache, cough, chest pain and dyspnoea; radiographic findings of lymphadenopathy are often found with one or more areas of pneumonitis. A higher incidence of disseminated cryptococcosis and cryptococcal meningoencephalitis was observed in blood cultures, tracheal aspirate studies and cerebrospinal fluid studies, both accounting for 31.1% of the total, 28.5% had invasive aspergillosis and 6% had histoplasmosis.

.3 HOSPITAL STAY OF PATIENTS WITH SYSTEMIC MYCOSIS/VIH TREATED WITH ANF-B IN THE INFECTIOUS DISEASES HOSPITAL 2015 - 2017

ICU STAY/DAYS (grouped)

		Frequency	Percentage	Percentage valid	Cumulative percentage
Valid	<= 10	82	54,3	54,3	54,3
	11+	69	45,7	45,7	100,0
	Total	151	100,0	100,0	

Table 3 ICU STAY IN ICU PATIENTS WITH MYCOSIS/HIV INFECTOLOGY HOSPITAL YEAR 2015 - 2017
SOURCE: HOSPITAL OF INFECTIOUS DISEASES STATISTICS DEPARTMENT AUTHOR: MICHELLE SOLÓRZANO RONQUILLO

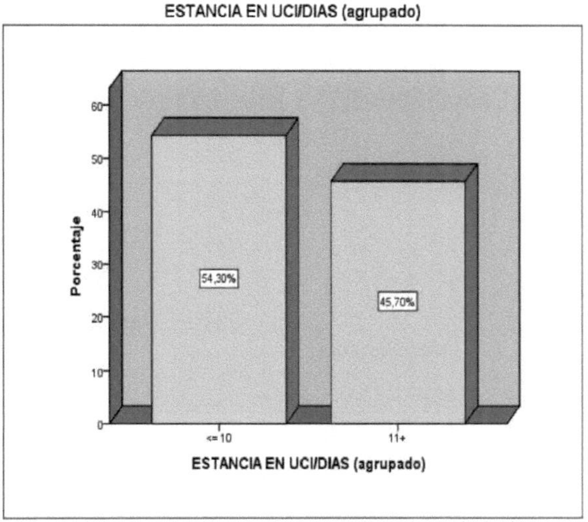

Illustration 3 ICU STAY IN ICU PATIENTS WITH MYCOSIS/HIV
INFECTOLOGY HOSPITAL
YEAR 2015 - 2017

Analysis: The most frequent reason for admission of patients with medical illness to the intensive care unit is acute respiratory failure requiring mechanical ventilation, which occurs in more than 30% of cases. Although it is true that mortality in this type of patient has been decreasing in recent years, we can observe that 54.3% of patients with systemic mycosis and HIV who were treated with amphotericin B spent less than ten days in hospital, 45.7% of patients spent less than eleven days in intensive care.

.4 ADVERSE EVENT AND AGE

Cross table ADVERSE EVENT AGE

		AGE				
		<= 25	26 - 42	43 - 58	59+	Total
EVENT ADVERSE	HYPERKALIEMIA	0	1	13	4	18
	HYPONATHROMIA	1	5	8	2	16
	INSUFFICIENCY ACUTE LIVER DISEASE	5	7	27	6	45
	NEPHROTOXICITY	2	16	22	10	50
	NOT REGISTERED	3	5	11	3	22
Total		11	34	81	25	151

Table 4 ADVERSE EVENT AND AGE OF PATIENTS
SOURCE: INFECTOLOGY HOSPITAL STATISTICS DEPARTMENT
AUTHOR: MICHELLE SOLÓRZANO RONQUILLO

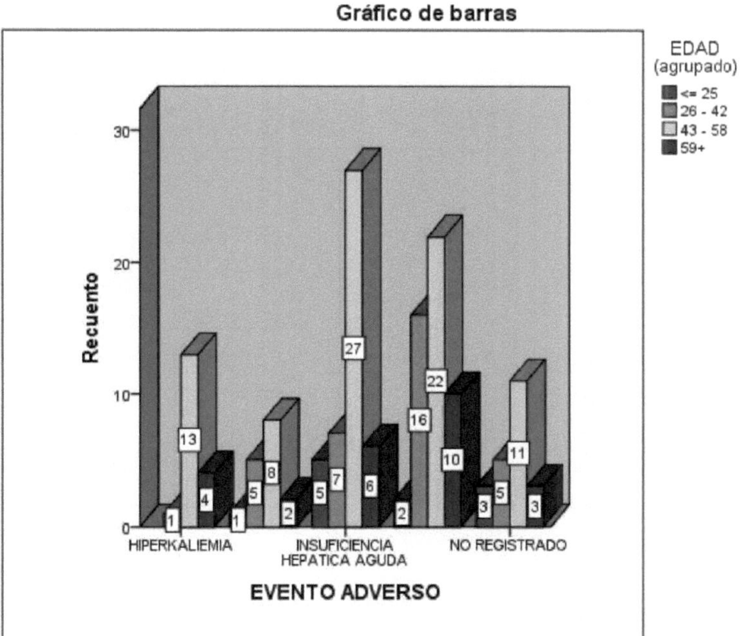

Illustration 4 ADVERSE EVENT AND AGE OF PATIENTS

In this table, age groups were established and correlated with the adverse events recorded in the group of patients under study, we can see that of the 50 cases of patients with nephrotoxicity, it is observed that there is a higher frequency of these events in the group of patients between 43 - 58 years old, where 22 cases were recorded; we also show that there are 45 cases of patients with liver failure; it is shown that 27 cases were recorded in the group of patients between 43 and 58 years old.

.5 ADVERSE EVENT AND SEX OF PATIENTS

Cross-tabulation ADVERSE EVENT SEX

Count

		SEX		Total
		FEMALE	MALE	
ADVERSE EVENT	HYPERKALIEMIA	11	7	18
	HYPONATHROMIA	10	6	16
	ACUTE LIVER FAILURE	23	22	45
	NEPHROTOXICITY	28	22	50
	NOT REGISTERED	11	11	22
Total		83	68	151

Table 5 ADVERSE EVENT AND SEX OF PATIENTS SOURCE: INFECTOLOGY HOSPITAL STATISTICS DEPARTMENT AUTHOR: MICHELLE SOLÓRZANO RONQUILLO

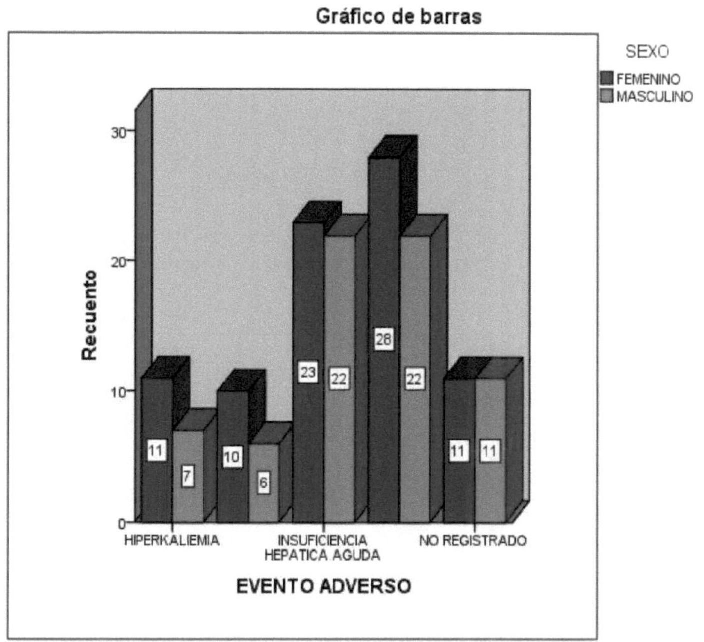

Illustration 5 ADVERSE EVENT AND SEX OF PATIENTS

It shows that there was a higher frequency of cases with adverse events in female patients, with 28 female patients with nephrotoxicity; 23 patients with acute liver failure, 11 female patients with hyperkalaemia; of the 57 cases of male patients with adverse events, 22 were due to nephrotoxicity, 22 with acute liver failure, 7 patients with hyperkalaemia and 6 male patients with hyponatraemia.

.6 DISTRIBUTION BY AGE GROUP OF PATIENTS WITH

SYSTEMIC MYCOSES/VIH INFECTIOUS DISEASES HOSPITAL OF INFECTIOUS DISEASES PERIOD 2015 - 2017

AGE (grouped)

		Frequency	Percentage	Percentage valid	Cumulative percentage
	<= 64	130	86,1	86,1	86,1
Valid	65+	21	13,9	13,9	100,0
	Total	151	100,0	100,0	

Table 6 DISTRIBUTION BY AGE GROUPS OF PATIENTS WITH SYSTEMIC MYCOSIS/HIV SOURCE: HOSPITAL OF INFECTIOUS DISEASES STATISTICS DEPARTMENT AUTHOR: MICHELLE SOLÓRZANO RONQUILLO

Within the distribution of the 150 patients analysed in this study we can observe that 86.1% of the total were under 64 years of age; patients over 65 years of age had a cumulative percentage of 13.9%.

.7 GENDER DISTRIBUTION OF PATIENTS WITH SYSTEMIC MYCOSES/VIH HOSPITAL OF INFECTIOLOGY PERIOD 2015 - 2017

		Frequency	Percentage	Percentage valid	Cumulative percentage
Valid	FEMALE	83	55,0	55,0	55,0
	MALE	68	45,0	45,0	100,0
	Total	151	100,0	100,0	

Table 7 SEX DISTRIBUTION OF PATIENTS WITH SYSTEMIC MYCOSIS/HIV SOURCE: INFECTOLOGY HOSPITAL STATISTICS DEPARTMENT AUTHOR: MICHELLE SOLÓRZANO RONQUILLO

The distribution of patients registered with systemic mycosis and HIV who were treated with amphotericin B is shown: 55% were female patients and 45% male patients, with a higher incidence of mycosis in female patients.

- DISCUSSION

The unit of analysis was the medical record and patient information was collected in the statistics department and included all patients who were on amphotericin B treatment due to microbiological diagnosis or clinical suspicion of systemic mycosis and who had amphotericin B administration recorded on the prescription.

Amphotericin B is considered the treatment of choice for severe fungal infections. However, its administration is associated with adverse reactions, mainly nephrotoxicity, which sometimes hinder its use. The incorporation of amphotericin B into lipid infusions has been reported to decrease its toxicity, but the reason for this phenomenon has not been fully elucidated. It has been suggested that this effect may be due to slowing of the passage of amphotericin B into tissues.

A total of 151 patients were identified in the 24-month period under analysis. The average age of the patients was 64 years, ranging from 18 to 76 years, with a female predominance (n=83;55%). Among the HIV seropositive patients, the most relevant fungal infection was cryptococcal meningoencephalitis (n=47;31.1%) and invasive aspergillosis (n=43;28.5%). in 39 patients who received amphotericin B at the Clinical Hospital of the University of Chile in 2009, where the average age of the patients was 45 years (range 18-76 years) with a predominance of males (n=22; 66.7%); five cases presented infection by Candida spp (12.8%), five possible and one proven cases by Aspergillus sp (15.4%), four by C. neoformans (10.3%) and one case of mucormycosis (2.6%) (20).

In this study, the most frequently reported adverse reaction was nephrotoxicity (n=50;33.1%); similarly, in the study by Quinteros et al. in 2009, nephrotoxicity developed in three of 32 treatments (9.4%) in which monitoring of renal function was available. Nephrotoxicity was only observed among patients with previously normal renal function and no patient required dialysis directly caused by the drug (20). This study also recorded that 22.5% of patients included had hydroelectrolytic disorders, recorded with potassium disorders such as hypokalaemia (potassaemia<3.5 mEq/L) compared to the study by Quinteros et al in which hypokalaemia occurred in eight treatments (21.6%). (20)

The purpose of this study was to provide more information on its indications, forms of use, adverse reactions associated with the use of this drug and the outcome of the patients treated. To this end, a retrospective study was designed to include a larger number of patients with various underlying pathologies, both critical and less severe, with different aetiologies, and thus obtain a representative picture of the scenario of the use of this compound and its complications. This series enrolled 150 patient treatments over two years of follow-up.

CHAPTER V

• CONCLUSIONS AND RECOMMENDATIONS

.1 CONCLUSIONS

The objectives are met:

- The Hospital de Infectologia de Guayaquil provides 90,000 outpatient, inpatient and emergency care visits per year, attending an average of 7,000 patients per month; the incidence of adverse drug reactions to amphotericin B per year is estimated at 47 new cases per 100 patients with systemic fungal diseases.
- Of the patients who met the inclusion criteria (HIV patients with systemic mycoses), the use of amphotericin B resulted in adverse reactions in 85.4% of all cases.
- A higher incidence of disseminated cryptococcosis and cryptococcal meningoencephalitis was observed in blood cultures, tracheal aspirate studies and cerebrospinal fluid studies, both accounting for 31.1% of the total, 28.5% had invasive aspergillosis and 6% had histoplasmosis.

- The median age of HIV/systemic mycosis patients who experienced adverse drug reactions due to the use of Ampho-B was 65 years.
- It is recorded that 55% were female patients and 45% were male

patients.

- The average length of hospital stay was 10 days per patient.
- Adverse drug reactions recorded were Nephrotoxicity (33.1%), Acute Liver Failure (29.8%), Hyperkalaemia (11.9%) and Hyponatraemia (10.6%).

.2 RECOMMENDATIONS:

- Monitoring of hepatogram, electrolytes and renal function should be done every 24 hours in patients receiving amphotericin B infusion in the critical care area.
- Drug dosage should be adjusted in all patients with chronic kidney disease and liver failure, consider rotating antibiotics in case of intolerance.
- Initiate empirical treatment with amphotericin B in suspected cryptococcal meningoencephalitis in HIV-positive patients until culture results are available.

CHAPTER VI

BIBLIOGRAPHY

1. Baddley J. Diagnosis and treatment of invasive pulmonary aspergillosis in HIV-infected patients. J Clinic. 2015.

2. Denis G. Relevance of the EORTC criteria for the diagnosis of invasive aspergillosis in HIV-infected patients, and survival trends over a 20-year period in France. Clin Infect Dis. 2015;(p 46:183).

3. Gonzalez M. Analysis of liposomal amphotericin B use. Revista Iberoamericana de micologia. 2016;: p. 109 - 113.

4. Spanish Journal oh Chemotherapy. Liposomal amphotericin B: 20 years in Spain. Revista Quimioterapia. December 2016;:: p. Pages 1 - 31.

5. Torrado S. Pharmaceutical development of amphotericin B polyaggregate formulations. Complutense University of Madrid. 2015.

6. Catalán M. Systemic antifungals. Pharmacodynamics and pharmacokinetics. Rev Iberoam Micol. 2015.

7. Jimenez Q. Liposomal amphotericin B in the treatment of systemic fungal infections in the neonate. An Esp Pediatr. 2014.

8. Ponton S. Amphotericin B Lipidococcus Complex: Results of the application of a use criteria. Farm Hosp. 2015;: p. 161 - 164.

9. CifUentes T. Hepatotoxicidad por Farmacos/ Drug-induced hepatotoxity. Rev Clin Med. 2016;: p. Vol 3. no.3 50-57.

10. Calderon C. Drug-induced nephrotoxicity. Journal of the medical students of the industrial university of Santander. 2017;: p. (8) 45-51.

11. Banchero P. Drug-induced agranulocytosis. Scielo Journal - Uruguay. 2015;: p. (14) 65-78.

12. Schaffner E. Administration of amphotericin B as a 24-hour infusion compared with 4-hour administration reduces nephrotoxicity and other adverse effects without reducing efficacy. Elsevier. 2015;: p. 15.

13. Wood. Undiagnosed tuberculosis in a community with high HIV prevalence: implications for tuberculosis control. Am J Respir Critic Care Med. 2011.

14. Bernardo. Diagnosis of pulmonary tuberculosis in HIV-uninfected adults. UpToDate. 2015.

15. Robb. Prospective study of acute HIV-1 infection in adults in East Africa and Thailand. N Engl J Med. 2016; 374(2120).

16. Peterman B. Kaposi's sarcoma among people with AIDS. Lancet. 2015.

17. Cox G. Clinical manifestations and diagnosis of Cryptococcus neoform meningoencephalitis in HIV patients. www.uptodate.com. 2017;: p. 134 - 146.

18. Wang Y. Innate immune evasion strategies against cryptococcal meningitis caused by Cryptococcus neoformans. med int infect. 2015 .

19. Argentine Society of Infectious Diseases. Current role of amphotericin B deoxycholate in oncohematological patients. Committee on Infections

in Immunocompromised Patients. 2014.

20. Roxanna Quintero AFNA. Use of amphotericin B deoxycholate and its adverse reactions in a university hospital in Chile. Hospital Clínico Universidad de Chile, Santiago Servicio de Farmacia (RQA) Departamento de Medicina (CNM, CGA. 2012;: p. 27 (1): 25-33.

21. Department of Health and Human Services. Panel on Antiretroviral Guidelines for Adults and Adolescents. Guidelines for the use of antiretroviral agents in HIV-1-infected adults and adolescents. 2014.

22. Denis G. Relevance of the EORTC criteria for the diagnosis of Invasive Aspergillosis in HIV-Infected Patients, and Survival Trends over a 20-year Period in France. Clin Infect Dis. 2015;: p. 46:1813.

23. Sax P. Acute and early HIV infection: clinical manifestations and diagnosis. 2018 June.

24. Dansinger. Practice Guideline: Identification, Assessment and Treatment of Overweight and Obesity in Adults. www. nhlbi.nih. gov/guideline s/obesity/prctgd_c.pdf. 2013.

25. National TB Center. Radiographic manifestations of tuberculosis: a primer for clinicians, 2nd edition. NTBC. 2010.

26. to BBe. Pulmonary Aspergillosis: An alternative diagnosis to lung cancer after positron emission tomography. Thorax. 2011;: p. 66:638.

27. Fortún J. Clinical forms and treatment of aspergillosis. Elsevier. 2012; 3(34-46).

28. Johson. Pulmonary aspergillosis: An alternative diagnosis to lung cancer from positron emission tomography. Thorax. 2014;(66:638).

29. Kauffman C. Epidemiology and clinical manifestations of invasive aspergillosis. New Eng Med. 2015;(355 - 377).

30. Lopez R. Amphotericin B: Determination in various biological fluids by liquid chromatography. Med Int Infec. 2015 Barcelona - Spain;: p. 129.

31. MOH. Guia de Atencion Integral para Adultos y adolescentes con infeccion por VIH/SIDA. Guia practica clinica MSP. 2016.

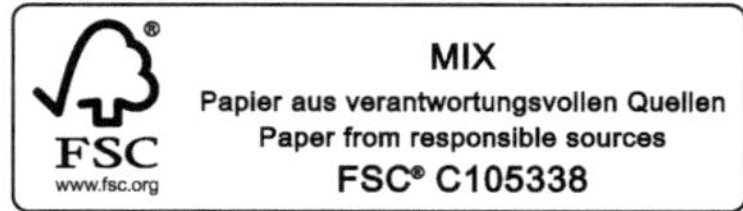

Printed by Books on Demand GmbH, Norderstedt / Germany